Healthful Minds:

A Guide to Alzheimer's Well-being

By

Winifred C. Brandon

Table of Contents

INTRODUCTION

Greetings and welcome to this comprehensive guide on Alzheimer's disease, a kind of mental road map to assist you navigate this complex mental illness. Consider it a journey through the many facets of how our brains function, particularly in the context of Alzheimer's disease.

We're going to discuss the early stages of Alzheimer's disease and when a person starts to experience cognitive confusion. But do not panic as we're keeping things lighthearted and casual, similar to a friendly discussion amongst friends.

This book functions as a kind of manual that covers both the scientific and interpersonal aspects of being there for one another. We're all part of this together, regardless of who is experiencing it or the people who are supporting them. Thus, let us explore the essence of Alzheimer's disease - simple, comprehending, and infused with a hint of optimism.

The difference between dementia and Alzheimer's

Despite their frequent interchangeability, these phrases have distinct meanings. Dementia is not a particular illness. It's a general word that covers a broad spectrum of symptoms. The capacity of persons to carry out daily tasks independently is impacted by these symptoms. Typical dementia symptoms include:

A reduction in memory

Modifications in cognitive abilities

Inadequate decision-making and reasoning abilities

Reduced attentiveness and focus

Alterations in language

Alterations in conduct

In terms of dementia, Alzheimer's disease is the most prevalent. Alzheimer's is a degenerative illness that progressively impairs memory and other critical mental abilities.

Memory and other critical mental functions are gradually lost due to the degeneration and death of brain cell connections and the cells themselves, but this is not the sole effect. Dementia has a wide range of forms and causes, such as:

Lewy body dementia [LBD]

Frontal lobe dementia

Vascular dementia

TDP-43 encephalopathy associated with limbic predominance and aging

Traumatic encephalopathy that persists

Dementia due to Parkinson's disease

The disease Creutzfeldt-Jakob

The disease Huntington's

Mixed-type dementia

Alzheimer's disease is a particular type of brain disease, but dementia is a broad phrase. It is characterized by dementia symptoms that worsen over time. Early indications of Alzheimer's disease frequently include problems in memory, thinking, and reasoning abilities since the disease initially affects the area of the brain linked to learning. The symptoms worsen with time and include disorientation, behavioral abnormalities, and other difficulties.

Alzheimer's disease early warning signs

Regular forgetfulness can sometimes be mistaken for Alzheimer's disease. You should be aware that while forgetfulness can play a significant role in the early stages and symptoms of Alzheimer's disease, there is much more to this condition.

First, you often worry and wonder whether you are getting Alzheimer's when you meet someone and suddenly forget their name or when you have stored your keys somewhere secure and can't remember where you put them.

The truth is that memory lapses happen frequently, particularly to those who lead hectic lives with obligations to their families and jobs and are constantly consuming a ton of information from tablets, laptops and mobile devices.

Not every random forgetfulness or memory loss indicates Alzheimer's disease. You should be aware too, that memory loss is one of the initial symptoms of Alzheimer's for the majority of sufferers. They can particularly struggle to remember recent occurrences and pick up new knowledge. As Alzheimer's disease worsens, memory loss becomes more and more disruptive to day-to-day activities. The individual could:

Forget someone's name or struggle to find the appropriate word in a conversation

Ignore the latest discussions or incidents.

Get lost on a well-known route or at a familiar location.

Forget about anniversaries and appointments.

Lose items they kept somewhere

Alzheimer's patients often experience memory loss as one of their initial symptoms, but they might also experience issues with other cognitive functions including reasoning, thinking, perception, or communication.

They could struggle with:

Language, making it difficult for them to follow a discussion or to repeat themselves

Visual skills: difficulty estimating distance or recognizing items in three dimensions; increased difficulty climbing stairs or parking

Having trouble focusing, planning, or organizing—having trouble deciding, coming up with solutions, or completing a series of activities (like preparing a meal)

Orientation: the state of being disoriented or forgetting the time of day.

Alzheimer's disease usually has minor initial symptoms, but as time goes on, they get more severe and begin to interfere with day-to-day activities. Take prompt action if you believe you are forgetting things more than usual and there are additional dementia-related symptoms. Alzheimer's disease symptoms include gradual declines in thinking, reasoning, and memory, as well as daily disruptions in memory.

Hey, though, hold on.

That appeared to be an easy question with an easy response.

Nevertheless, before you act on anything this book suggests, here's what you should know:

Since each person with dementia is different, no two will experience dementia symptoms in precisely the same manner.

A person's personality, overall health, and social circumstances all play a significant role in deciding how dementia affects them.

Thus, while the symptoms of Alzheimer's disease and other forms of dementia differ, they all share many general characteristics. The most typical symptoms are loss of practical abilities and memory, which can cause disengagement from social or professional activities. You should speak with your doctor if you believe that these issues are interfering with your everyday life or the lives of someone you know.

Make your diagnosis as soon as possible, but don't jump to conclusions.

Seven phases of Alzheimer's disease

The most prevalent type of dementia, a term used to characterize the loss of cognitive function, is Alzheimer's disease. Alzheimer's disease can eventually make it difficult to do everyday tasks like dressing and conversing.

Understanding the symptoms of each stage of Alzheimer's might help you support the person you care about in managing their illness.

Recall that each person's experience with Alzheimer's varies. Since the stages are merely supposed to be guidelines and often overlap, it can be challenging to pinpoint which stage your loved one is in. The timing and severity may vary for each individual.

Stage 1: In the Absence of Symptoms

Alzheimer's-related brain alterations start before symptoms become apparent, just like with many other diseases.

This phase, which is also referred to as "pre-clinical Alzheimer's disease," probably starts ten or fifteen years before any symptoms appear. This pre-clinical stage has no known treatment at this time. Since the likelihood of developing Alzheimer's disease rises with age, it's critical to maintain routine primary care visits so that screening can identify the disease's early symptoms. Your loved one may be moving into the second stage of Alzheimer's if you see a decline in their cognitive ability.

Stage 2: Basic Forgetfulness

Everyone has occasional forgetfulness, and as people age, this is likely to happen more frequently. Alzheimer's disease can appear to be typical aging forgetfulness in its very early stages. Your loved one may still be able to drive, work, and interact with others despite memory lapses that include forgetting people's names or where they put their keys. But these forgetfulness episodes increase in frequency. You'll likely become aware of this before your loved one does, which could allow you to intervene early and stop the disease's growth.

Stage 3: Notable Memory Problems

Age will no longer be the primary cause of the noticeable changes that individuals experience throughout this era. At this point, a person's everyday routine starts to become increasingly disturbed, hence diagnosis rates are high.

This stage is characterized by common challenges beyond name forgetfulness and object misplacing. Your loved one might:

Experience memory problems with previously read books or periodicals

Find it harder to remember plans and to organize things.

Find it more difficult to recall a term or name

Face difficulties at work or in social situations

Your loved one may experience more worry during this stage, and some may even want to downplay their problems. While these emotions are common, waiting to consult a doctor will simply make the symptoms worse. Discussing treatment choices, including medication and care planning, with your loved one's doctor is the best way to manage symptoms.

Stage 4: Memory Loss and Beyond

At this point, brain injury frequently affects cognitive abilities other than memory, such as difficulties with language, organizing, and math. Your loved one may find it more difficult to carry out everyday duties as a result of these issues.

This phase, which may extend for several years, will cause your loved one to struggle greatly with memory. They could still be able to recall important information about their past, such their marital status or state of residence. Their recall of events that happened a long time ago will typically be far superior to their recollections of everyday things like what they saw on the news or a conversation they had earlier in the day.

Additional difficulties at this point include:

Unsure about the time of day and their location

Higher chance of getting lost or straying

Alterations in sleep habits, such as sleeping during the day and being restless at night

Having trouble dressing appropriately for the occasion or the weather

Being in social situations or other circumstances requiring a lot of thought can be quite frustrating during this time and moodiness or withdrawals are prevalent. Your loved one may also have other personality changes as a result of the brain damage, such as becoming cynical about people, losing interest in activities, or experiencing depression. Medications can often help with these kinds of symptoms.

Stage 5: Reduction in Self-Sufficiency

Your loved one might have had little trouble living alone up to this point. They were able to get by without your regular help, but you did occasionally stop by to see how they were doing.

During this phase, it's possible that your loved one would struggle to recall significant others, including friends and close family. Basic duties like dressing themselves could be too much for them, and they might have trouble learning new things.

At this phase, emotional shifts are also typical and include:

Hallucinations: Perceiving nonexistent things

Delusions: Irregular thoughts you take for granted

Paranoia: believing that people are against you

Stage 6: Extensive symptoms

Being independent means that you have to be able to react to your surroundings, such as knowing what to do when the phone rings or the fire alarm goes off. For those with Alzheimer's disease, this gets challenging during stage 6. At this point, your loved one's symptoms will be more severe, making it harder for them to handle their own care and making them more dependent on others.

It could also get hard to communicate at this point. Even when your loved one is still able to speak, it can be difficult to talk about certain ideas, such where they are hurting.

There may still be notable alterations in personality, such as heightened anxiety, delusions, hallucinations, and paranoia. Your loved one can grow angrier with you as their level of independence declines. You can talk to your care team about behavioral techniques and medications that could be helpful in these situations.

Even though some patients may not experience the aforementioned behavioral changes and remain happy during the course of their illness, when they do, one should keep in mind that they are not conscious of what they are doing at this time, so try not to take it personally.

Stage 7: Inability to Exercise Physical Control

Alzheimer's disease eventually results in significant mental and physical damage because it kills brain cells. Your loved one's body can start to shut down as their mind finds it difficult to communicate and assign responsibilities.

This is where your loved one's needs would really start to rise. For assistance with walking, sitting, and eventually swallowing, they might require 24-hour care.

As a result of their decreased movement, they may also be more susceptible to diseases like pneumonia. Keep their lips and teeth clean, apply antibiotic ointment to cuts and scrapes promptly, and make sure they have their annual flu vaccination to help prevent illnesses.

Now that you are aware of your loved one's Alzheimer's stage, what should you do?

It's crucial to understand the extent of Alzheimer's disease dementia, but that's just the first step. With this information, you can make sure your loved one is receiving the care they require and interact with their doctors more effectively.

Additionally, by obtaining medical supplies like a wheelchair, learning symptom management techniques, or being ready for additional support like an assisted living facility, you'll be able to make ready for whatever comes next.

Primary cause of Alzheimer's

It is believed that aberrant protein accumulation within and around brain cells is the root cause of Alzheimer's disease. Amyloid is one of the proteins involved; deposits of this protein encircle brain cells in the form of plaques. The other protein is known as tau, and deposits of it cause tangles in brain tissue.

Scientists now know that this process starts many years before symptoms manifest, even if the precise cause is unknown.

A reduction in the chemical messengers, or neurotransmitters, that are responsible for conveying signals or messages between brain cells occurs when brain cells are impacted.

People with Alzheimer's disease have particularly low levels of the neurotransmitter acetylcholine in their brains.

Different parts of the brain shrink with time. Memories are typically the first areas to be damaged.

Different parts of the brain are affected in less common forms of Alzheimer's.

Rather than memory issues, the initial symptoms might be issues with vision or language.

Enhanced risk

There are a number of established risk factors for Alzheimer's disease, even if the exact cause of the illness is still unknown.

Age

The single most important aspect is age. After age 65, your chance of getting Alzheimer's disease increases every five years. Nonetheless, Alzheimer's disease is not limited to the elderly. One in twenty persons who have the illness are younger than 65. This type of Alzheimer's disease, also known as young-onset or early-onset Alzheimer's disease, can strike people as early as age 40.

Family background

Though the actual increase in risk is tiny, the genes you inherit from your parents can increase your risk of acquiring Alzheimer's disease.

However, Alzheimer's disease is brought on by the inheritance of a single gene in a small number of families, and the likelihood of the illness being handed down is significantly higher.

If multiple family members have experienced dementia throughout the years, especially in their early years, you might want to consider genetic counseling to learn more about your risk of Alzheimer's disease in later life.

The Down syndrome

The risk of Alzheimer's disease is increased in those who have Down syndrome.

This is due to the fact that the genetic alterations that result in Down syndrome can also eventually contribute to the accumulation of amyloid plaques in the brain, which in certain cases can result in Alzheimer's disease.

Head injury

A head injury has been linked to an increased risk of dementia in the future. When playing sports, wear a helmet, fasten your seat belt and "fall-proof" your home to protect your brain.

Heart-head connection

The strongest evidence connects heart health and brain health. This relationship makes sense as the heart is in charge of pumping blood to the brain via one of the body's largest networks of blood arteries, which supplies nutrition to the brain.

Many disorders affecting the heart and blood arteries seem to enhance the risk of acquiring Alzheimer's or vascular dementia. Heart disease, diabetes, stroke, hypertension, and excessive cholesterol are a few of these.

Extensive evidence supporting the heart-head relationship comes from studies conducted on donated brain tissue. According to these researches, the presence of strokes or blood vessel injury in the brain increases the likelihood that plaques and tangles may result in Alzheimer's symptoms.

One way to lower your risk is to:

Give up smoking

Consuming a balanced, healthful diet

Living a physically and mentally active life

Reducing your weight if necessary

Reducing alcohol consumption

As you age, getting regular health examinations

Additional danger indicators

The most recent studies also points to the importance of other factors, albeit this does not imply that these factors are directly to blame for dementia.

Among them are:

Loss of hearing

Untreated depression (although Alzheimer's disease symptoms can also include depression)

Loneliness or social isolation

A sedentary lifestyle

Could Alzheimer's also afflict young people?

Those who assert that Alzheimer's disease cannot affect young people lack knowledge. In actuality, only roughly 5% of those who get Alzheimer's disease experience symptoms while they are younger. Therefore, at least 200,000 Americans have an early onset variant of Alzheimer's if 4 million Americans suffer from the illness. Early onset refers to the early onset of Alzheimer's disease. No, my intention is not to frighten you but to raise awareness of Alzheimer's disease's early beginning and how it can affect young people as well.

Indeed, early-onset Alzheimer's is a rare type of dementia that affects people at a younger age than the majority of Alzheimer sufferers. The reason behind the early beginning of Alzheimer's disease in these individuals is unknown to experts; nonetheless, the majority of researchers propose that early onset Alzheimer's patients suffer from a form of the disease known as "familial Alzheimer's disease". They probably have Alzheimer's since they were raised by parents or grandparents who also got the disease when they were younger.

Three genes—the APP, PSEN 1 and PSEN 2, which differ from the APOE gene that can raise your risk of Alzheimer's in general—have been related to early onset Alzheimer's disease that runs in families. Less than 1% of instances of Alzheimer's disease overall and between 60 and 70% of cases with early onset are shared by these three genes.

Alzheimer's disease may manifest before the age of 65 if you carry a hereditary mutation in one of these three genes. For medical reasons, a precise diagnosis of early-onset Alzheimer's is essential in order to rule out other possible conditions and obtain the best treatment possible for both personal and professional reasons. Thus, begin implementing precautions right away. Don't put off adopting a healthy lifestyle till you are sixty years old. Move quickly.

Ways for preventing Alzheimer's

Millions are afflicted with this mostly preventable disease called Alzheimer's. In your thirty's, it may begin to take shape.

The most intriguing fact, though, is that just about 1% is inherited. 99% of it is under your control, contrary to what you may believe.

Thus, the following actions can be taken to avert one of the most severe and terminal illnesses in the world:

There are eight things to be aware of:

1. Consume a low-GL diet (glycemic load; I'll explain).

2. Consume good fats for the brain.

3. Consume B-complex foods

4. Consume antioxidants

5. Consume probiotics to maintain intestinal health.

6. Work Out

7. Maintain mental acuity

8. Take a nap

Alright, let's simplify this:

A "low GL diet": what is it?

In essence, it stabilizes blood sugar levels.

Alzheimer's risk is often doubled in people with type 2 diabetes.

In other words, replace white bread, pasta, and rice with brown ones and cut back on sugar and carbohydrates for a simple victory.

Next up, nutritional supplements

2. Good fats for the brain (Omega 3s and vitamin D)

Your brain is essentially as vital as it gets because it is composed of 90% fat, of which 60% is DHA omega 3.

You should definitely supplement your diet unless you frequently consume a lot of algae/seaweed or oily seafood. As for vitamin D, the majority of us are deficient in it. Furthermore, sources can be found outside as well as everywhere.

3. Vitamin B

Omega 3 supplements have been shown to have a significant synergistic effect with B vitamins, which are fantastic for brain function. If all else fails, supplements that combine Omega 3s and B vitamins are the bare minimum you need.

4. Antioxidants

They lessen inflammation and offer protection from oxidants, which are harmful to the brain and more prevalent as people age.

The winners are strawberries, bilberries, and blueberries.

5. Consume probiotics to maintain intestinal health.

This is significant since your mood and mental health are greatly influenced by the health of your gut because it is the site of communication between your brain and neurotransmitters like serotonin, dopamine, and GABA.

Adopt probiotics; this is a must.

6. Work Out

It simply means moving on a regular basis; nothing crazy here.

It has been demonstrated that walking for 10 to 40 minutes a day significantly enhances brain function (the closer to 40 minutes, the better results you obtain).

Move now to preserve your life.

7. Maintain mental acuity

Truly, the saying "Use it or lose it" applies.

Play games like chess, sudoku, and languages; converse with friends; read other people's viewpoints; and make a daily effort to keep your mind active.

8. Take a nap

Since those who experience high levels of stress, worry, despair, or other mental health disorders are more likely to acquire Alzheimer's disease, this is really about rest, sleep, and finding meaning in life.

Thus, you safeguard your brain for the future by maintaining mental health today. Does that make sense?

Although completely incurable, Alzheimer's disease can be largely avoided.

How?

Consume wholesome vitamins, exercise, get enough sleep, and maintain mental clarity.

It's not that difficult.

As you get older, you should start to take it more seriously. In your 30s, you can dismiss it.

Foods to avoid Alzheimer's

Would you like to eat the appropriate foods to prevent the two most horrible aging diseases known to man? This chapter will teach you what kinds of foods to eat as you age so that you don't develop dementia or Alzheimer's.

Making sure you have enough choline in your diet is the greatest way to avoid dementia and Alzheimer's disease. Male adults should take at least 550 milligrams of choline daily, according to the NIH, whereas female adults only need to take 425 milligrams. So why is choline such a big deal? A vitamin called choline is vital to the health of the brain. A 2019 study that was published in the American Journal of Clinical Nutrition found that consuming more dietary choline lowered your risk of cognitive deterioration. Furthermore, a 2019 study headed by Arizona State University researchers came to the same conclusion about choline's ability to fend against Alzheimer's. In light of all of this, the following ten foods are the best in preventing dementia and Alzheimer's disease:

1. Beef liver

Up to 355.5 mg of choline can be found in a normal slice of beef liver. For men, that already accounts for 65% of their daily choline requirements, and for women, it may reach 84%. This is best enjoyed as a pan-fried slice with olive oil.

2. Eastern oysters

Eastern oysters in a 12-ounce can have up to 220.3 mg of choline in them. For men, that equates to 40% of the daily intake, and for women, to 52%. A delicious way to savor this is to combine it with a hot bowl of creamy chowder.

3. Breast of chicken

Lean chicken breast weighing six ounces has 198.9 mg of choline per serving. That represents 47% of a woman's daily requirement for choline and 36% of a man's. Although there are many other ways to prepare chicken breast, roasting it in the oven with some herbs is one of the most common methods.

4. Legs of chicken

Chicken legs contain roughly 180.6 mg of choline per leg, which is richer than chicken breast but still helps against dementia and Alzheimer's disease. 42% of women's daily requirements and 33% of men's are already met by eating a leg with skin. Baste it with soy sauce and bake it in the oven for a tasty meal.

5. Salmon

Each piece of salmon has a slightly different amount of choline. For instance, a six-ounce portion of farmed Atlantic salmon contains 153.9 milligrams of choline, whereas a plate of sockeye salmon contains up to 191.4 mg. However, 122.4 mg of choline from wild coho salmon will boost brain function as well. Salmon can provide you with at least 22% to 29% of your daily requirement for choline, regardless of the species.

6. Chops of pork

Pork chops' choline level varies according to the amount of fat they contain. Choline content in lean pork chops is lower than that of fat chops. Choline concentration varies depending on the type of pork chop; a six-ounce lean drop has 152.8 mg, while a six-ounce fattier chop has 167.7 mg. Whatever your choice, you would receive at least 36% of your daily requirement for calcium if you're a woman and 28% if you're a guy.

7. Cod

One filet of Atlantic cod normally has 150.7 mg of choline. That makes up 27% of a man's daily need for choline and 35% for women. Coating this fish in olive oil and baking it with cherry tomatoes and lemon slices is one of the greatest ways to eat it for optimal brain health.

8. Eggs

One of the foods highest in choline density is eggs. There are normally 146.9 mg of choline in one egg. That is equivalent to 27% of a man's daily requirement for choline and 35% for a woman. The ideal way to eat eggs is soft-boiled because excessive heat damages the choline and eggs.

9. Lean ground beef

Ground beef is a flavorful and excellent source of choline, regardless of how it is prepared. For instance, 6 ounce patties made of ground beef that is 97% lean will provide you with around 146.2 mg of choline. That is roughly 27% of what men and women need each day and 34% of what women need.

10. Roasted ham

A couple of regular roasted hams have 136.5 mg of cholesterol. This corresponds to roughly 32% of the daily needs for women and 25% for men. One of the finest ways to cook this for optimal brain support is to add it to scrambled eggs to increase the amount of choline even further.

Including these routines in your diets would be beneficial whether or not you have a family history of dementia and Alzheimer's disease. By doing this, you can promote good brain health and lower your risk of developing cognitive decline as you age.

Ways to assist a loved one suffering from dementia or Alzheimer's

Seeing a loved one suffer from dementia is frequently confusing and painful.

They could become angry and confused, repeat themselves, or forget where they are. They will require care from someone as memory diseases deteriorate brain and nervous system cells over time. They may also change the way they think, talk, and behave. Perhaps a day will come when people fail to recognize you.

We refer to it as "the long goodbye." Even while cutting-edge new drugs may be able to slow the advancement of Alzheimer's disease, being prepared can help you support your loved one with dignity during those years.

See your loved one for who they truly are.

It is unnecessary and may even be counterproductive to correct them every time they say or believe something incorrect.

It will only anger and perplex them to bring up the friend's death if they believe they will be seeing them for a poker party ten years ago. Also, it's likely that they'll forget in a few minutes.

What does it achieve? It's possible that they are incapable of understanding. Your reality is not the same as theirs.

Participate or switch the subject.

The Alzheimer's Association advises using basic, direct, calm communication in a quiet area with little distractions. This involves asking yes/no questions one at a time and maintaining eye contact. In addition, you can be more engaged by using visual and tactile cues like touch or pointing.

Honor their wishes.

Talk to your relative about their financial wishes and end-of-life care preferences as early as possible in their sickness, while they are still capable of making decisions. Respect their wishes completely.

They still have the freedom to live their lives as they see fit, even if they have Alzheimer's. Did they hang out with buddies all the time? Set up frequent weekly or monthly get-togethers with one or two pals. Were they fond of sweets? Therefore, don't give up all sweets. Replace them with more wholesome fruits and vegetables.

A memory issue can make losing one's independence one of its most difficult aspects. The secret is to understand their pre-illness lifestyle.

Try to keep up with familiar activities that your loved ones with Alzheimer's enjoyed when you visit or care for them.

Patients with dementia initially lose short-term memory.

Alzheimer's patients frequently misplace household or personal belongings, including glasses, or forget crucial appointments and duties when the condition is first developing. Families can assist by providing cues, such as labeling cupboards, drawers, and doors to indicate what's inside and using calendars to record mealtimes, doctor visits, medication schedules, and bill due dates.

While these more recent memories are blocked by neurological disorders, older memories can reappear.

People occasionally turn back to the past because that is what they can easily access. They may try to go back to that previous existence in an effort to "make sense of the world," since their home and loved ones appear unrecognizable and different from what they recall.

Call to Schedule

Keep an eye out for any safety hazards.

Dementia patients are more likely to be involved in catastrophic, life-threatening collisions, particularly if they become disoriented or drive when very unwell. The Alzheimer's association estimates that 60% of persons with dementia wander at least once and more frequently.

Keep an eye out for telltale symptoms like restlessness and difficulty recognizing familiar places—avoid crowded places like malls. Families ought to establish a strategy for emergencies, which can involve signing up for a roaming response service.

The National Institute on Aging emphasizes in its home safety checklist that any dangers, including car keys, matches, prescription drugs, power tools, alcohol, plastic bags, and firearms, should be removed or securely locked away. Later phase Dysphagia, or difficulty swallowing or chewing food, is another common complication of Alzheimer's disease that can lead to choking. Talk to their doctor as soon as you or anybody else observes them coughing during meals.

There are often mood swings.

Communicating can be difficult for Alzheimer's sufferers, particularly if the disease progresses to the intermediate or advanced stages. Hence you won't always be able to tell if they're depressed, hungry, exhausted, bored, or having trouble eating. Anger can surface when you try to make them do something they don't feel well enough to do or when their needs aren't addressed. If they're depressed, look into what's causing it and try to find some relief, like more sleep or snacks.

Assure them of your safety and do the thinking for them.

A phenomena known as "sun-downing" occurs when some Alzheimer's patients become agitated or even violent in the evenings. For those who are unprepared, this might be alarming. The cause is not entirely clear. Hormones, circadian rhythms, dread of shadows in the dark, or recollections of nighttime events may all be connected to it.

Families who follow a regular daily schedule that incorporates socialization and adequate exercise might reduce suffering. Experts advise turning on the lights early and reducing stimulation and activity (TV, loud noises, large meals, or long showers) as the day comes to an end.

The emotional cost of a "long goodbye" is high, regardless of whether you're the primary caregiver or a worried family member, especially when it gets more difficult for you to get in touch.

Make sure you're taking care of yourself in addition to your loved one.

CONCLUSION

Let's take a moment to consider the insights we have received as we draw to a close our exploration into the world of Alzheimer's. Being aware of this complicated issue is the first step toward empathy.

Alzheimer's is a powerful enemy, but with the right information, encouragement, and compassion, we can overcome its difficulties.

Let this serve as a reminder that the journey is far from over as we close this chapter. You are an important part of the story of Alzheimer's, whether you are looking for information, providing assistance, or just spreading awareness. Together, with empathy, understanding, and a common goal for a time when memories are treasured and minds are embraced with kindness, let's continue this journey.